A Short History of Psychiatry

A Short History of Psychiatry

By Frederick Lyman Hills

LM Publishers

"Forth from my sad and darksome cell,
Or from the deep abyss of hell,
Mad Tom is come into the world again
To see if he can cure his distempered brain."

— *Old Tom O'Bedlam Song, XVII century.*

Psychiatry:
Ancient, Medieval and Modern.

Among the achievements of the nineteenth century none surpass the revolution wrought in the field of psychiatry. The care of the insane today excites the interest not only of philanthropists and alienists, but of all right-minded men and women. "No reflecting mind," says Letchworth, can be indifferent to the question of making proper public provision for the treatment and care of those afflicted with an insidious disease from which no measure of intellectual or physical strength or worldly prosperity affords any certain immunity — a disease, which, prone to feed upon excitement, finally transforms the noblest faculties of our race into a wreck so appalling that in its contemplation the human intelligence becomes bewildered and dismayed. At no time in the history of civilization has the importance of this subject been more thoroughly acknowledged; and probably at no time have influences contributory to mental derangement been more powerful than they are today." It is eminently profitable at this time to review the treatment of the insane in ancient days, to recall the misfortunes of the unhappy madman during the dark ages of history, and to note the gradual evolution of the psychiatric science of today.

Going back into the very dawn of history we find scattered references to the treatment of madness, which was looked upon as a punishment by the gods or ascribed to demoniacal possession. The earliest known historical reference to insanity occurs in Egyptian papyri of the fifteenth century B, C. In one of these, according to Mahaffy, music is spoken of as employed in the treatment of insanity, and many formulæ are given for the cure of diseases caused by an evil spirit dwelling within the body.

Probably the next earliest record is that found in Hebrew history, referring to the same therapeutic agent, this time used to calm the troubled spirit of Saul (1055 B. C). In the first book of Samuel we read: When the evil spirit was upon Saul, that David took a harp and played with his hand; so Saul was freshed and was well and the evil spirit departed from him." The legendary history of Greece affords numerous instances of madness, but as to the treatment in these early times there is only eloquent silence.

The belief in demoniacal possession was prevalent among all primitive peoples, furnishing a clue for such treatment as was anywhere at- tempted, and this belief, giving way a few centuries later to a partial realization of the physical basis of insanity in the best medical minds, recurs again in the darkness and decadence of the middle ages but magnified and rendered terrible by the ignorance and gross superstitions of the time. In ancient Egypt, demons were exorcized and lunatics purified in temples dedicated to Saturn. The god Khons is said to have answered prayers for the cure of an Asiatic princess. The priests of Egypt, who were also physicians of the day, were not un- mindful of the benefit of hygienic measures and combined with them the charm of music and the influence of the beautiful in nature and in art.

No reference is made in the literature of antiquity to places set apart for the care of the insane.

In Greece they were sometimes cared for by the priests in the temple of Aesculapius. More often they were detained at home by their friends if dangerous, or allowed, if mild, the freedom of the country unrestrained and unmolested. Many of the soothsayers, sorcerers and sibyls of these days were undoubtedly insane, and the mental condition of some was known to those who sought their offices. Restraining devices were generally used in all violent forms of madness. Herodotus relates that Cleomenes (519-491 B. C), king of Lacedaemon, becoming insane, was imprisoned by his kindred and his feet put in the stocks. While so bound he asked the man left to watch him for a knife. This being refused he began to threaten the man, who, becoming frightened, gave him the knife and he at once made repeated gashes in his limbs and abdomen until he died.

In the time of Euripides (480-406 B. C.) it would appear from his account of the madness of Hercules that madmen were bound with cords and fastened to the nearest convenient spot. Hippocrates, the Father of Medicine (460-377 B. C), described three forms of mental disease and seems to have recognized alcoholic insanity. He was the first to lay stress upon the physical basis of insanity and ridicules the treatment given by the priests. He used phlebotomy, purgatives, emetics, baths, a vegetable diet, exercise, music and travel.

He regulated the use of hellebore, a drug held in high esteem from the dawn of history. Writing to Democrates he said: "Hellebore when given to the sane, pours darkness over the mind, but to the insane it is very profitable." This drug was believed to act powerfully in cleansing and invigorating the intellectual faculties. It is said that Carniades, the Academic, when preparing to refute the dogmas of the Stoics, went through a course of purgatives by hellebore.

Melampus, son of Amythaon, is said to have cured the daughters of Proetus, King of Argos, of melancholy, by purging them with hellebore. According to tradition Melampus had observed that the goats who fed on this plant were purged, and having administered it to the king's daughters, who were wandering in the woods under the delusion that they were cows, he cured them and received the hand of one of them in marriage and a part of the kingdom of Argos as his reward.

So celebrated was this medicinal agent as a mental remedy that the poets of antiquity sang its praises. Horace, in allusion to the 'happy madman,' says:

> He, when his friends at much expense and pains, Had amply purged with hellebore his brains. Came to himself — "Ah, cruel friends!" he cried, "Is this to save me? Better far had died Than thus be robbed of pleasure so refined, The dear delusion of a raptured mind."

Persius thus addresses Xero in his fourth satire, telling him to relinquish the arduous duties of government:

> "Thou hast not strength, such labors to sustain. Drink hellebore, my boy—drink deep and purge thy brain."

Hippocrates had his patients collect this medicine themselves at Anticyra, in Thessaly, and thus made its use an incident of a very hygienic course of treatment. In cases of suicidal melancholia he employed mandragora, first spoken of by him in the treatment of this disease.

The attitude of the state toward the care of the insane at the period soon after the death of Hippocrates is thus expressed by Plato (375 B. C.) in *'Laws of the Republic'*: "If anyone is insane, let him not be seen, openly in the city, but let the relatives of such a person watch over him at home in the best manner they know and if they are negligent let them pay a fine."

The teachings of Hippocrates and his followers were probably the guide for those who had to do with the insane during the next two centuries, and nothing further appears in medical literature until the careful study of insanity made by Asclepiades of Bythinia (100 B. C). He distinguished between illusions and hallucinations, noted the changing mental states of individual cases and made some innovations in the treatment. He recommended his patients to be placed in the light rather than confined in dark rooms or cells, disapproved of venesection, and of the fomentations of poppy, mandragora or hyoscyamus. He prescribed abstinence from food, drink and sleep in the early part of the day; the drinking of water in the evening; that gentle friction should be employed and, later on, liquid nourishment should be ad-ministered and the friction repeated.

By these means it was his hope to induce sleep. Themison, his disciple, prescribed a more liberal diet, baths and astringent fomentations. Another of his disciples recommended stripes in the treatment of the insane, but it is doubtful if this was sanctioned by the master. Asclepiades also attempted substitutive medication, advising intoxication in the general treatment of insanity.

Celsus (A. D. 5) formulated wise rules for the hygienic and moral treatment, but unfortunately advised also the use of hunger, chains and chastisements to subjugate the patient. He would have those scolded whose mirth was excessive and resort to torment should conciliation fail.

To startle a patient suddenly, to terrify him, this was excellent. But he directed that all things possible should be done to divert the melancholy and to excite cheerful hopes. Pleasure should be sought in fables and in sports, in music and in reading aloud. To quiet the excited and to favor sleep, he made use of a rocking motion and the sound of a waterfall.

Aretaeus (A. D. 80) gave a detailed description of mania and melancholia, considering the latter to be the incipient stage of the former. Little is known as to his methods of treatment, except that he does not mention restraint in his descriptions.

Galen (A. D. 150), the celebrated advocate of the humoral pathology, gives little as to treatment, but his theory of insanity is interesting. Moisture, he says, produces fatuity, dryness sagacity, and therefore the sagacity of a man will be diminished in proportion to the excess of moisture over dryness. Therefore preserve a happy medium between these opposite qualities, use venesection if you think the whole body of the patient contains melancholy blood. Bleeding must be avoided if madness arise from idiopathic disease of the brain.

Then follows Coelius Aurelianus (A. D. 195), leaving a most remarkable treatise on the treatment of insanity, preaching gentleness and humanity, skilled attendance and non-restraint. He thus ex- presses himself regarding the physicians who resort to harsh methods of treatment: "They seem rather to lose their own reason than to be disposed to cure their patients, when they liken them to wild beasts who must be tamed by the deprivation of food and the torments of thirst. They go so far as to counsel bodily violence and blows, as if to compel the return of reason by such provocations, a deplorable method of treatment that can only aggravate the patients' condition, injure them physically, and offer to them the miserable remembrance of their sufferings whenever they recover the use of their reason." He taught that the patient should be put in a quiet room, moderately warm and light, excluding everything of an exciting nature. The bed should be firm and fixed to the floor and should have a straw mattress.

The attendants should be carefully instructed. "If the sight of other persons irritates them and only in very rare instances, restraint by tying may be employed, but with the greatest precaution, without any unnecessary force, and after carefully protecting all the joints and with especial care to use only restraining apparatus of a soft and delicate texture, since means of repression employed without judgment increase and may give rise to furor instead of repressing it." He used fomentation by applying warm moist sponges over the eyelids to relax them and influence the circulation in the membranes of the brain. He advised emollient and astringent applications, the latter made of galls, alum, etc., soothing and invigorating poultices, baths of oil and natural hot baths. He denounced abstinence and ordered a full diet.

He spoke against the practice of making the patient intoxicated, the use of hellebore, of aloes and of venesection. During convalescence he recommended farming, walking, riding, singing and theatrical entertainments. In the latter scenes of a solemn and tragic character were to be enacted to guard against excitement.

With the passing of Galen and Coelius Aurelianus the sun goes down into the black clouds of ignorance succeeding the fall of the Roman Empire; and the lunatic is left to drag out a miserable existence, generally neglected and alone throughout the dark centuries following, to and through the middle ages.

There is a fitful gleam faintly illuminating the scene momentarily as when Alexander of Tralles (A. D. 560), or Paulus Aegineta (A. D. 630) reiterates the teachings of Aurelianus, but they lay stress more upon the medicinal than the hygienic treatment and are forgetful of his admonitions against chains and imprisonment.

The earliest hospital for the insane known was founded in Jerusalem in the fifth century as a refuge for anchorites whose minds became affected through their penances.

The middle ages are defined by Hallam as dating from the invasion of France by Clovis at the end of the fifth century to the invasion of Naples by Charles VIII at the end of the fifteenth. During the first half of this period there seems scarcely to have been any intellectual or political development.

The whole of Europe was, almost without exception, sunk in the darkest ignorance and the most wretched barbarism. In some countries the awakening was earlier than in others, but the darkness did not anywhere die out at once. As gradually the clouds began to lift and the signs of returning light were here and there discernible only a fraction of a special class, a limited portion of the clergy, were in any way affected, and the mass remained for long bound down by servility, ignorance and superstition. "The struggle among the races for the possession of the countries that had been loosed from the Roman yoke," says Sibbald, "'continued for centuries to make the state of war persistent and almost universal."

When not in conflict with their neighbors, the constant friction and strife within the individual states still prevented organization and natural development. "In such a state of society little thought could be bestowed on anything which did not directly relate to the fierce struggle for very life in which every state and every individual was engaged." There was no time for philanthropy, for the care of the suffering, for the relief of the poor, for comforting the sick in body or mind. Slowly the leaven of

Christianity was at work, a silent force effecting slow but deep-rooted changes in the constitution of society, beginning about the eleventh century to gradually bring about the abolition of slavery and exerting an influence in instituting some sort of provision for those whose mental condition was thought to be the result of disease.

The monks were also the physicians during the dark ages and the monasteries offered quiet retreat and seclusion for many insane, together with sympathy and protection which could not be found elsewhere. Spiritual agencies were everywhere popularly believed to be most efficacious in the cure of madness, and many and long were the pilgrimages made to the shrines of those saints who were believed to have special influence over the mentally afflicted, and many miraculous cures were said to have been brought about through exorcism and prayer. There were many wells through Europe and the British Isles, each with its particular saint, to which the insane were brought to bathe and to pray.

At St. Nim's Pool in England, it was the custom to plunge the patients backwards into the water and drag them to and fro until their excitement was subdued. If they showed signs of recovery thanks were offered in a neighboring church, but if not, the treatment was continued until no hope remained. From the seventh century even to the present day lunatics have made pilgrimages to the shrine of St. Dymphna at Gheel, and here the first colony for the insane originated through a slow process of evolution, and stands today as the best representative of the community or family system of caring for the insane.

So great a part did superstition and religious bigotry play in the treatment of insanity that the estate of the lunatic grew ever worse. Any man who exhibited anything unusual in conduct or language was at once suspected by his neighbors of necromancy or commerce with the Devil and looked upon with suspicion. Any manifestation of peculiar genius, the display of inventive ability or promulgation of a new doctrine rendered a man liable to torture, imprisonment or death. The belief in demoniacal possession, and witchcraft, was distinctly recognized in the Bible and fostered by the church.

All over Europe persons undoubtedly insane were burned or hanged as witches or were whipped in the public squares to drive out the evil spirits. Pope Innocent VIII. in 1488 appointed inquisitors in every country armed with apostolic power to find and punish those of whom he thus declared: "It has come to our ears that numbers of both sexes do not avoid to have intercourse with the infernal fiends, and that by their sorceries they afflict both man and beast. They blight the marriage bed; destroy the births of women, and the increase of cattle, they blast the corn in the ground, the grape in the vineyard, the fruit of the trees, and the grass and herbs of the field."

Thus stimulated by the church the search for persons punishable for these crimes was everywhere successful. It is probable that one-fourth of the 40,000 persons executed for witchcraft during the first eighty years of the seventeenth century in England alone were insane. Among the thousands of persons tortured, burned and hanged as heretics there were doubtless many who, infected by surrounding fanaticism and carried away by exceptional beliefs, were really the victims of mental disease.

Persons afflicted with the more quiet forms of insanity without excitement were often regarded as suffering in punishment for sin and were accordingly treated by fasting, pilgrimages and self-castigation. Some, the possessors of a certain shrewdness and drollery, were received into private houses and cared for, partly from charity, and partly because of the amusement to be derived from their eccentric speech and conduct. The conditions were practically the same in all European countries with the exception of Italy and Spain, where insane asylums were established during the latter part of the middle ages.

The Mohammedans preceded the Christians in the establisliment of asylums for the insane, and it is probable that as early as 1300 A. D. this form of charity was general in Mohammedan countries. A writer of the seventh century notices the existence of several such institutions at Fez. The asylum in Cairo was founded in 1304 A. D. Whether or not the Christians obtained the idea of the organization of such asylums from the Mohammedans, it is of interest to note that they are first found in Europe among those nations nearest to the Mohammedans and most subject to their influence.

To Spain is due the honor of establishing the first asylum in Christian Europe for the care of the insane exclusively. This was opened in Valencia in 1409 A. D. by a monk, Juan Gilaberto Joffre, who was moved by com- passion on seeing maniacs driven through the streets by hooting crowds of men and boys.

The treatment in these early establishments amounted to little more than seclusion and restraint, though the monks in charge of the asylum at Saragossa, established in 1425 A. D. had some conception of a rational open air treatment. Asyhmis were also opened at Seville and Valladolid in 1436 A. D. and at Toledo in 1483 A. D. "Two other very honorable facts may be mentioned," says Lecky, "establishing the preeminence of Spanish charity in this field. The first is that the oldest lunatic asylum in the metropolis of Catholicism was that erected by the Spaniards in 1548. The second is, that, when at the close of the eighteenth century, Pinel began his great labors in this sphere, he pronounced Spain to be the country in which lunatics were treated with most wisdom and most humanity.'"

In the twelfth century madmen were taken to St. Bartholomew's in London and, according to the monkish narratives many wonderful cures were effected.

Up to the sixteenth century monasteries and prisons and ecclesiastical hospitals contained cells into which lunatics were received, but it is probable that they were given little care or treatment and that the public at large was the chief beneficiary by their incarceration. In 1547 the first lunatic asylum not under ecclesiastical administration was established in England. The priory for the order of St. Mary of

Bethlehem founded by Simon Fitzmary, a sheriff of London, in 1247, in St. Botolph's without Bishopsgate, Lon- don, had for a century and a half been used for the reception of lunatics.

In this year the institution, for long before called Bedlam, was transferred by Henry the VIII to the authorities of the city, with an order that it be converted into a house for the reception of lunatics. It stood in an out of the way place, close to many common sewers and accommodated but fifty or sixty patients.

For very many years, however, the place remained a 'horrible prison,' says Sibbald, 'and not a hospital in any sense of the word.' "Up to the year 1770 the patients were exhibited to the public like wild beasts in cages, on payment of a penny, and they are said to have afforded much sport to the visitors who flocked to see them in numbers estimated at not less than 48,000 annually.

Some whose condition was so ameliorated that they were no longer considered dangerous to the public were licensed to go begging. On their left arm was placed an armilla—an iron ring for the arm about four inches long, which they could not get off." "They wore about their necks," says Aubrey, as quoted by Disraeli, "a great horn of an ox in a sling or bawdry, which when they came to a house they did wind; and they put the drink given them into this horn, whereto they put a stopple." In a Tom of Bedlam song which dates from the first part of the seventeenth century, the comforts of his asylum life are thus alluded to by the licentiated beggar:

> In the lovely lofts of Bedham
> In stubble soft and dainty,
> Brave bracelets strong.
> Sweet whips ding dong,
> And a wholesome hunger plenty.

About 1675 when the licensing of beggar lunatics was stopped by law, a new Bedlam three times the capacity of the old was erected in Moorfields, the necessity for increased accommodations becoming greater 'as the country came more and more into systematic government and as the wholesale burning of such unfortunate persons as wizards or witches died out.'

Little appeared in medical literature during this period upon the care of the insane. Daniel Sennert (1572-1637) wrote sensibly upon mania and melancholia, but left nothing as to treatment, except to bleed and to purge. Sydenham (1624—1689) had little to say on mental affections. An adherent to the current doctrine, he attributed insanity to a disabling of the 'animal spirits' by a prolonged fermentation. He prescribed a cordial of Venice treacle, containing the flesh and broths of vipers, amber and sixty-one more ingredients in Canary wine and honey to be given three times a day, the patient to remain in bed and to be liberally supplied with liquids.

For ordinary mania he ordered the withdrawal of nine ounces of blood on two or three occasions with three days' interval between each bleeding.

A course of pills of colocynth and scammony followed, and on the days when the patient did not take the pills he was to have an electuary composed of conserve of monk's rhubarb, rosemary, candied angelica and other pleasant ingredients.

Something more rational was attempted in Paris when by an Act of Parliament in 1660 the insane passed through two wards, especially reserved for them in *Hotel Dieu*, the ward St. Louise for men containing ten beds for four each and two small beds; the ward St. Martin for women containing six large beds and six small ones. Treatment here was by means of douches, cold baths, repeated bleedings, hellebore, purgatives and antispasmodics.

If there was no improvement in a few weeks they were sent to the Petits Maisons, the Salpetriere or the Bicetre, where they were kept clothed in rags, confined by chains, poorly fed, bedded on rotten straw, often in cells infected with disease. As in England on holidays they were exposed to the gaze of the public, admitted for a small fee as to a menagerie.

In 1667 Dennis, in Paris, successfully employed transfusion of blood taken from a calf in the case of a young man insane after an unhappy love affair.

The early years of the eighteenth century saw the gradual evolution of the asylum idea and the slow increase in the number of establishments for the insane, founded not only by the state but by private individuals. The condition of the insane in the latter was particularly distressing for many years, and, even until well on in the last century, many of them were more to be dreaded than the larger public asylums.

Dean Swift had in mind the foundation of a hospital for the insane as early as 1731 when he wrote the verses on his own death and described his determination thus,

> He gave the little wealth he had
> To build a house for fools and mad;
> And shewed by one satiric touch,
> No nation wanted it so much.

This object he had afterward always in mind, and, although suffering much for several years and his mind finally becoming affected in 1742, he made plans for its establishment and, dying in 1745, left his whole property, about $60,000, for the founding of St. Patrick's Hospital in Dublin, which was opened in 1757 for the reception of fifty patients.

The methods of treatment employed in the middle of the eighteenth century are thus set forth by Dr. Richard Mead, physician to George II. in his "Medical Works" (1762). "Authors, both ancient and modern, recommend a great number of medicines, some which are suit- able to maniacal, others to melancholy patients; but both sorts agree in the property of correcting the bile, which is acrid at first, then be- comes viscid and black as pitch. Moreover the very blood in this disorder is thick, fizy and black. Now it will be observed that most of the medicines proper to be given in this disease are in some degree endowed with the property of opening and scouring the glands and in- creasing perspiration. Of this kind are the strong-smelling gums, specially asafoetida, myrrh, Russian castor, and camphire, which last is asserted to have an anodyne quality and to procure sleep with greater certainty and safety than opium. In melancholic cases chalybeats are also very proper. In fine, a frequent use of the cold bath is very serviceable, especially in maniacal cases. For nothing, as Celsus says, is of such benefit to the head as cold water." He cautions against the use of stripes or other rough treatment as unnecessary, binding alone being sufficient to restrain the maniacal, who ^are all cowards.' He attempted to stop the ill-timed fits of laughter of some by chiding and threatening; to dissipate the gloomy thought of others by music and such diversion as they formerly took delight in.

He cautioned the physician to attend carefully to the free action of the bowels and kidneys and instead of applying blisters to the head he says, "Better in imitation of the ancients to shave the head, and then rub it with vinegar in which rose flowers or ground-ivy leaves have been infused; and also to make a drain by passing a seton in the nape of the neck, which is to be rubbed with a proper digestive ointment and moved a little every day, in order to give a free issue to the purulent matter." He ordered slender diet, mostly of gruels and meats easy of digestion, disapproved of giving anodynes to procure sleep and recommended walking, riding, playing at ball, swimming and travel by land or sea in convalescence.

The latter part of the eighteenth century witnessed an awakening of the minds of men throughout the civilized and enlightened nations of the world to a realization of the man's duty to his fellow man.

The dissemination of knowledge among the people was gradually killing out the grosser forms of superstition, holding such a hypnotic influence over the ignorant. The spirit of liberty, fraternity and equality was abroad. With this zeal for the acquirement of knowledge, the spirit of investigation and the kindling of enthusiasm for scientific research, philanthropic ideas began to develop in men's minds, pity for the suffering and the unfortunate and a desire to better the condition of all. Prison reform was agitated, hospitals were organized for the sick in body.

The treatment of the insane was made a matter for legislative investigation and although little or nothing was done toward the immediate relief of their condition, yet public sentiment was being slowly aroused in their behalf. Gradually the light of a brighter day was dawning. The propriety of abusive treatment, of cruelty, of chains, of stripes, formerly regarded as essential for the control of the maniac, or looked upon with indifference, was now brought into question. Much was written relative to insanity during this period but no decided step was taken for the betterment of conditions until near the close of the century when the noble-hearted Tuke, in England,

and the brave Pinel, in France, started the grand reform, broke the fetters and brought the great restorative, hope, to stimulate the weakened mind.

The York Asylum, founded by general subscription in 1777, for 'the decent maintenance and relief of such insane persons as were in low circumstances' was, about 1791, the worst among the bad institutions in England. In this year a young woman, a member of the Society of Friends was committed to the York Asylum. Her friends were denied the privilege of seeing her and in a few weeks she died. Her death arousing suspicion of improper treatment among the Friends, one of their number, Mr. William Tuke, "resolved (1792) to establish an institution in which there would be no secrecy and where the patients would have humane and judicious care." Thus was the

Retreat at York established and, in 1796, launched upon its memorable career, continuing from the first a leader in psychiatric progress.

The year 1792 also is made memorable by the appointment of Philip Pinel as physician to the insane at the *Bicetre*. Coming to this position a trained alienist, he was deeply stirred by the condition of the men confined there, fifty of them in chains, many for a long period of years. His repeated and persistent appeals to the Commune for authority to release them from their bonds were finally given a reluctant affirmative answer, and in the end he was able to remove the chains from all the patients and to continue the good work at the *Salpetriere*, an institution exclusively for women.

Turning now to our own country we find the care of the insane in the American colonies prior to the Revolution to differ in no way from the treatment during the same period in Europe. In the Old Colony Laws of Plymouth (1660) provision was made that persons who commit suicide "shall be denied the privilege of being buried in the common burying place of Christians, but shall be buried in some common highway, where the selectmen of the town where such persons did inhabit, shall appoint, and a cartload of stones laid upon the grave, as a brand of infamy, and as a warning to others to aware of the like damnable practice."

In jails, almshouses and the outhouses of private dwellings, the insane were kept, often in chains and in filth, and deprived of light and proper warmth. No attempt was made toward special provision for them until 1745, when an asylum was erected in New York City, on the spot where the City Hall now stands, for the reception of the 'indigent poor, the sick, the orphan, the maniac and the refractory.' But the first institution in America for the remedial treatment of the insane was founded in 1751 in connection with the Pennsylvania Hospital. Being opened 1752, "it was," says Kirkbride, "for a long period of years far in advance of all other receptacles for the insane in the United States, and, having the advantage of physicians like Bond, Shippen, Push, Wister, Physick and others of equal ability, its wards were constantly filled, and its advantages eagerly sought by patients from the most distant parts of the Union."

It is noteworthy that, besides Dr. Thomas Bond, of Philadelphia, and Benjamin Franklin, the Society of Friends was active in the inception of this hospital, a society later to be influential in the establishment of the York Retreat in

England and the Friends Asylum at Frankfort, Pa. (1813), showing in these early times a more enlightened philanthropy than any other religious body and giving the impetus to a movement which in the early years of the nineteenth century was to effect a revolution in the treatment of the insane.

The first governmental institution in America was erected by the province of Virginia at Williamsburgh in 1773; but it was not until the era of peace and quietude following the wars of the Revolution and of 1812, and after the successful inauguration of the state governments that public sentiment became thoroughly aroused to the necessity of better care for these unfortunates, and state institutions sprang into existence.

During the thirty years following the war of 1812 twenty-three public and private asylums were opened in the United States.

The treatment at this time was largely influenced by the writing of Dr. Benjamin Rush, a man of great intelligence and benevolence whose 'Observations on

Diseases of the Mind' (1812) contained much of value as to the moral treatment of the insane, but who was behind Pinel in realizing the advantage of kind treatment and the harmfulness of restraint. "A prevailing error found in his writings on insanity," says a writer in the "^American Journal of Insanity' (Vol. 4) "is that the insane are to be disciplined and governed, that those who have the care of them must obtain dominion over them by fear or by other means that we may think improper." He says that the physician on entering the chamber of the deranged person should first 'catch his eye and look him out of countenance.' After trying many ways to obtain obedience he says, "If these prove ineffectual to establish a government over deranged persons, recourse should be had to certain modes of coercion."

Among them were the straight jacket, the tranquilizing chair (invented by a Dr. Darwin and consisting of a stout post revolving on a pivot and bearing a chair into which the patient was bound in the longitudinal position when a sedative effect was desired or in an erect position to secure intestinal action), the withdrawal of pleasant food and pouring cold water down the coat sleeves. "If all these modes of punishment should fail of the intended effect," he adds, "it will be proper to resort to the fear of death."

But the man who did more than any other, probably, to forward the humane care of the insane, was Esquirol, who succeeded Pinel at the *Salpetriere* in 1810. Devoting himself with zeal and with singleness of purpose to this ministration, he brought about still greater reforms in the housing, the regimen and medical care of the insane, and in 1817 gave the first course of lectures ever delivered on insanity. These were largely attended every year by physicians from all countries.

He traveled through France investigating everywhere the condition of the insane, arousing the interest of the magistrates and, through his reports to the superior authorities, causing the abolition of many abuses and much misery. He saw ten asylums opened in France and the insane taken from 'their narrow, filthy cells, without light and air, fastened with chains in these dens,' in which he found them, and placed in asylums where the use of chains was abandoned, where walks and gardens were accessible, and where beds and good food were provided and the attendants did not go 'armed with sticks and accompanied by dogs.'

The same spirit of progress was now abroad in every enlightened country of Europe and in America. Asylums were built, treatises upon mental medicine became more numerous, classification of mental disease and more careful clinical studies were attempted, societies were organized for the study of insanity and periodicals appeared whose pages were given wholly to the discussion of psychiatric subjects and the propagation of the new doctrines.

"In the period which elapsed from 1830 to 1850," says Letchworth, "'great and rapid advances were made throughout the United States in methods of caring for the insane. The reforms then accomplished attracted the attention of Europe, and it may be said, without any egotism, that they were in advance of contemporary progress in other countries." Much of this reform was due to the exertions of Dorothea L. Dix, who about 1837 began a career of remarkable success in arousing public attention and securing legislative action for the betterment of the condition of the insane. She is said to have been influential in the establishment of thirty-two asylums for the insane. But unfortunately this high standard of achievement was not maintained.

During the civil war and the early period of reconstruction this reform suffered a reaction, and the country failed to keep pace with the progressive movement in other lands. Within the last thirty years of the century, however, rapid advance was made, and today the standard of work done for the insane in America is not lower than that attained in other countries.

The period of large and imposing buildings, palatial in exterior appearance, has passed. The buildings erected twenty or thirty years ago were uniformly massive, three- or four-story structures, the interiors often monotonous and cheerless. Today the tendency is to place the patient in surroundings as cheerful and homelike as possible.

To have smaller buildings, comfortably furnished, with pictures on the walls, with books, games and the means for light amusements and employment. No longer is the patient forced to pace ceaselessly long cheerless corridors, the walls lined with benches and heavy chairs and bare of all adornment.

Now, instead of large blocks of buildings, the modern hospital consists of a group of cottages, best of two stories, separated or connected by a low corridor. Here the patients are separated into small groups carefully classified as to their mental condition. These buildings are surrounded by nicely kept grounds, with green lawns dotted with shrubbery and flowers.

There are groves to afford a shady retreat, and here the patients spend much time every pleasant day. Many of them have the parole of the grounds and come and go without oversight. Freedom is allowed as far as is consistent with safety. In many places the usual iron gratings have been removed from the windows and doors left unlocked.

But the institutions for the insane of today are not places merely of detention. The insane asylum, except for the chronic cases, in most states both here and abroad, has passed away and in its place has arisen a hospital to which the patient comes as a sick man to have the kind care and systematic treatment that the word hospital implies.

He is received and cared for by nurses trained to the work and is at once impressed with the idea that he is a sick man, so regarded by his fellow men, if not cognizant of it himself, and that he is to have done for him what careful nursing, hygienic surroundings and medical science can do. The perfection to which this system has attained varies much in different states; but all are tending to the same end, and ere long the care of the acute insane in all enlightened lands will be based upon the same scientific plan.

At the present time in Europe and America there is great activity within the walls of the hospitals for the insane. The study of the individual patient is more thorough than ever before. Not only are his mental symptoms diligently watched and recorded, but a careful systematic examination of all his bodily functions is undertaken. For this purpose laboratories are equipped and men trained to microscopical and chemical analysis are being more and more employed to carry on the work. The study of the physiology and pathology of the nervous system is being assiduously pursued and recent epoch-making discoveries in tissue-staining have stimulated this work, causing almost a revolution in the theories of nervous action; and it would seem that a better understanding of the functioning of the central nervous system was dawning.

The defects of distant organs, of the blood vessels, the blood, the lymph and all abnormal bodily conditions, are known to often have a deleterious effect upon the nervous system and improvement in the mental condition to be coincident with their removal.

The physician and the surgeon, the neurologist, the psychologist, the chemist and the pathologist are all at work hand in hand with the alienist to cure him who is the unhappy victim of mental disease.

In the modern hospital such moral measures are brought into operation as the companionship of a kind and congenial nurse, cheerful environment, the use of the minimum amount of restraint consistent with safety and efforts to amuse and divert the attention of the patient away from himself and his troubles, the attempt to arouse an interest in some light employment and the suggestive influence of a hopeful spirit. The therapeutic effect of exercise, massage, hydrotherapy and electrical influence are all called into use, and the medical treatment is directed to any complicating disorder of the bodily functions.

No part is overlooked. The physical machine is restored as far as possible to working order in the hope that mental restoration will be the consequence. In a hospital thus conducted harsh or abusive treatment means the immediate dismissal of the offender.

The selection of an efficient corps of attendants is a matter of the greatest importance. Much improvement has been brought about by the establishment of training schools in hospitals for the insane with systematic instruction in the duties of the nurse.

In a large and well organized institution an attendant entering the school is in a position to obtain instruction of so much general usefulness in the treatment of the sick that the hospital benefits not only by the more efficient service rendered, but also by the attraction of a superior class of applicants for the positions. "Much has been accomplished in rescuing the insane from chains, gloomy cells and scourgings," says Letchworth, "but the measure of reform in their behalf will not be complete until there is no possibility of their being subjected to the humours of ignorant, unfeeling and incompetent attendants." That training schools are an efficient means of accomplishing this reform there can be no doubt.

A most notable advance in the treatment of the insane was the introduction of the system of non-restraint—the disuse of all mechanical devices for restraining the freedom of bodily movement. This was first demonstrated to be practicable by Mr. Gardner Hill at the Lincoln Asylum, England, in 1836, and Dr. Connolly put the system into full operation at Hanwell in

1840. At first ridiculed as "the freak of an enthusiastic mind, that would speedily go the way of all such new-fangled notions" it was bitterly opposed for years by the superintendents of the large county asylums of England, and to Dr. Connolly is due the honor of having demonstrated its practicability and of having overcome after a prolonged struggle the opposition and prejudice against it.

Men like Todd, Woodward, Butler, Ray—names memorable in the history of American psychiatry—were not unmindful of the remedial value of sympathetic and kindly treatment, and, while the controversy over non-restraint was waged abroad, were independently carrying out the same humane doctrine and conducting their institutions on the same 'enlightened principles of conciliation and kindness.'

At the present day the system of absolute non-restraint is more in vogue in England than here where the necessity for some form of restraining appliance is still maintained to exist in certain instances. But it is evident from the annual reports of the American hospitals that the use of restraint is lessening each year.

In some institutions it is entirely abolished; in all it is used to a very limited extent and only upon the order of the attending physician. The means of restraint employed consist chiefly of the canvas camisole to restrain the movements of the hands and arms, the canvas or leather muff for the hands and the use of a strong sheet fastened across the bed if the patient is not in a condition to be up and about the rooms. In place of the sheet the hands and the feet may be restrained while the patient is in bed by soft rolls of cheesecloth.

The most recent advance in the care of the acute insane is in the movement toward the establishment of psychopathic hospitals for treatment and for clinical and pathological research in or near the large centers of population. In this most advanced work Europe has taken the lead, and such hospitals have been in existence for some years in the university towns of Germany and Austria.

That at Giessen, opened in 1896, is thus described by Dr. Frederick Peterson, president of the New York State Lunacy Commission—"It is in the town of Giessen, near the other hospitals used for teaching purposes, adjacent to the pathological institute, and consists of ten or eleven cottages for 116 patients, in a beautiful garden. The central building contains pathological, chemical, microscopical, photographic and psychophysical laboratories, besides a mechanical workshop, clinical auditorium, library, and a dispensary or polyclinic for outdoor patients. The necessary administrative offices and rooms for the director and assistant physicians are also here. There are cottages for private cases, and for quiet, suicidal, restless, and disturbed patients of each sex. This is probably the most complete hospital of its kind in existence at the present time."

Although as yet in Great Britain and America this work has not received the attention it merits, a beginning is being made.

At Albany, New York, a pavilion has been opened in connection with the Albany General Hospital for the reception of the acutely insane, and in Michigan the last legislature passed an act to "Provide for the Construction of and Equipping of a Psychopathic Ward upon the Hospital Grounds of the University of Michigan."

In Boston and Philadelphia out-patient departments have been in successful operation for several years. There is no doubt but that the next few years will see the general opening of such hospitals and out-patient departments in the larger cities throughout the country.

Another movement that is ripening to fruition in America is that for the establishment of 'After-care Associations' for the protection and help of needy patients upon discharge from hospitals, recovered, but without means of support. This idea originated in Germany as far back as 1829, with Hofrath Lindpaintner, who organized in that year a 'Society of Patronage' which exercised a paternal care over, and rendered assistance to, such persons for a period of two years following their recovery. Such associations were later formed in France, and in recent years the system has been in general operation in Germany, France, England and notably in Switzerland.

The work of these organizations, the establishment of which in this country has already been discussed by the American Neurological Association, consists in finding proper homes and employment for discharged patients, maintaining a general supervision over them and offering such financial or other aid as may be necessary again to put them in the way of earning a livelihood.

In spite of all efforts put forth to cure the acute mental troubles a large percentage of the cases prove rebellious and drift into chronic states of mental deterioration. The patients do not die, but live in good bodily health with intellect dulled to the higher interests of life and sink slowly into incurable dementia. Other cases are marked from the outset by the stigmata of chronicity, being slow and insidious in development, and the disease is often fully established before the patient's friends awake to a realization of the event. These chronic classes of the insane require a specialized treatment, a home where they can be protected from the world and from themselves, where congenial occupation may be obtained, where a strict but humanely enforced control may be exercised over their conduct and where their lives may be lived in comfort and in peace. Until recent years all classes of insane have been cared for in large institutions where proper classification has been difficult or impossible and where the acute and cur-able cases have been in daily contact with the incurable and the demented.

Of late much effort has been made to overcome this objectionable state of thing by the establishment of colonies, where the chronic insane may live in small separated cottages scattered in groups over a large tract of land. Here the patients live in small groups or families under conditions more approximating home surroundings. The farm and industrial shops furnish the occupation so necessary to relieve the monotony of life and to counteract abnormal tendencies.

The little colony has its chapel and amusement hall, sometimes a store, and furnishes an environment in which a man may live in comparative comfort and with a reasonable degree of contentment. Such colonies are now quite numerous in Europe and America and seem to furnish ideal conditions for the care of the chronic and presumably incurable cases. In Scotland, Germany, Belgium, and to a limited extent in Massachusetts, a system is in operation with a fair degree of success in which selected chronic cases are boarded out in private families in the country districts while under the observation and control of a govern- mental bureau or commission.

It is unfortunately a fact that many of the chronic insane are still detained in almshouses and poor farms not only in this country but abroad.

Here they, who are the unfortunate victims of disease and not to be held responsible for their condition, are obliged to associate with paupers and criminals and are kept in a condition unworthy of the civilization of the twentieth century. The cruelty of a past age still lingers in many of these places, and not only do they suffer from the stigma of their associations, but are too often the victims of improper and insufficient attendance and are not strangers to bonds and chains.

But the grand work of emancipation is still going on, and en- lightened public sentiment is everywhere at work and the realization of a fuller charity is surely not long to be delayed.

At the beginning of the twentieth century we are on the threshold of a new era in the working out of this great problem, and the scientific and philanthropic spirits of the day are laboring together and energetically toward its ultimate solution.